This Occupational Therapist Journal Belongs To:

Made in the USA
Middletown, DE
07 November 2019

78126304R00073